ASTHMA DIET COOKBOOK

Delicious Anti-Inflammatory Recipes For Reducing Symptoms, And Boosting Respiratory Health

DR ELIAN GRIFFIN

DISCLAIMER

The nutritional recommendations and recipes in this book are meant solely for informative reasons. They are not meant to replace the counsel, diagnosis, or care of a qualified medical expert. If you have any doubts about a medical condition or dietary requirements, you should always see your physician or another trained healthcare expert.

All reasonable efforts have been taken by the author and publisher to ensure that the information contained in this book is correct as of the date of publication. Recommendations may alter, though, as medical knowledge is always changing. When using any of the recipes or instructions found here, the user assumes all liability and assumes no risk, whether personal or otherwise. People who have certain dietary requirements or medical issues should speak with a healthcare provider for personalized guidance. The given recipes are only ideas; you may need to adjust them to suit your own nutritional needs, tastes, and tolerances.

When you use this book, you agree to release the publisher, the author, and their representatives from any liability for any claims, damages, liabilities, costs, or expenditures resulting from your use of the book.

TABLE OF CONTENTS

ABOUT THE BOOK

Understanding the relationship between diet and asthma forms the cornerstone of this book, giving readers insights into how dietary choices can either exacerbate or alleviate symptoms. By outlining key principles of an asthma diet, the book empowers people to adopt dietary habits that support respiratory function and overall well-being. The Asthma Diet Cookbook is an essential resource for people managing asthma, emphasizing the profound impact of diet on respiratory health.

The identification of individual food triggers—which enables readers to identify particular allergens or substances that may exacerbate asthma symptoms—is at the heart of the book. Realistic dietary goals are stressed, encouraging long-lasting adjustments that easily fit into everyday life. Regular adherence to a healthy eating plan not only aids in the management of asthma but also provides wider health benefits, boosting vitality and energy levels.

The book explores the vital nutrients that are necessary for managing asthma, including omega-3 fatty acids, antioxidants, vitamins, minerals like selenium and magnesium, fiber, and the significance of staying hydrated through water consumption. It also covers foods to stay away from, including common allergens, processed foods with additives, high-sodium items, sugary drinks, and foods that are known to increase mucus production.

Weekly meal plans and shopping lists simplify grocery trips, while batch cooking tips and portion control strategies help maintain consistency. The book offers a wide variety of recipes catered to different meal times, from nutrient-packed smoothies and whole grain breakfast bowls to anti-inflammatory salads, hearty soups, omega-3-rich fish dishes, and dairy-free desserts. Practical guidance on meal planning and preparation is provided; readers can create asthma-friendly meals without stress.

Snacks and appetizers include nuts and seeds mixtures, fruit snacks, and energy bars that are suitable for people with asthma. Drinks that help relieve asthma symptoms include herbal teas and smoothies that are high in water content. Lifestyle suggestions include workout regimens, methods for reducing stress, ways to avoid triggers in the environment, and more.

Expert tips from healthcare professionals round out the comprehensive guidance, ensuring readers feel informed and supported in their journey toward better asthma management through dietary choices. After addressing common concerns and answering frequently asked questions, the book offers practical advice on managing asthma flare-ups, modifying diets for children with asthma, navigating social events, and clearing up misconceptions.

CHAPTER ONE

RECOGNIZING THE LINK BETWEEN DIET AND ASTHMA

An understanding of the relationship between diet and asthma entails realizing how certain foods and nutrients can either aggravate or relieve symptoms. For example, some foods have anti-inflammatory qualities that aid in reducing airway inflammation, while others may aggravate respiratory conditions or trigger allergic reactions.

It's crucial to understand that although diet cannot treat asthma, it can be very effective in managing its symptoms and enhancing respiratory health in general.

To start comprehending this relationship, it's useful to know which nutrients are good for people with asthma. Omega-3 fatty acids, which are found in fish and flaxseeds, have anti-inflammatory properties that can help control asthma symptoms. Antioxidants, like vitamins C and E, which are found in fruits and vegetables, also support lung health by preventing oxidative stress. Processed foods, on the other hand, should be avoided because they contain a lot of artificial additives and preservatives.

Keeping a food diary can help identify patterns and potential triggers. This individualized understanding enables people to make informed dietary choices that support their respiratory health.

Speaking with healthcare providers or dietitians can provide additional insights and customized recommendations to optimize the diet for asthma management. This is just one aspect of a comprehensive approach to the diet-asthma relationship.

IMPORTANT GUIDELINES FOR AN ASTHMA DIET

The mainstays of an asthma-friendly diet are anti-inflammatory foods, hydration, and a balanced diet. Anti-inflammatory foods like nuts, leafy greens, and fatty fish can help reduce airway inflammation.

Including a variety of fruits and vegetables guarantees a rich intake of vital vitamins and minerals that support overall health. An effective asthma diet also emphasizes reducing inflammation, supporting the immune system, and avoiding known triggers.

Asthma management requires a balanced diet that includes sufficient amounts of protein, carbs, and healthy fats. Whole grains, lean proteins, and healthy fats from avocados and olive oil supply the nutrients needed without causing inflammation.

Probiotics from fermented foods and yogurt also help to support gut health, which is becoming more and more understood to be important for immune system function and inflammation control.

Asthma sufferers can effectively manage their condition by adhering to these fundamental principles. Proper hydration is another important consideration. Drinking plenty of water helps keep mucus thin, making it easier to clear from the airways. Herbal teas and natural fruit juices can also be helpful, but it's imperative to avoid sugary drinks and sodas, which can contribute to inflammation and weight gain.

RECOGNIZING INDIVIDUAL FOOD ALLERGENS

A vital first step in controlling asthma with diet is determining one's triggers, which can vary from person to person and require careful observation and documentation of individual responses to various foods. Common triggers include dairy products, processed foods, and certain additives such as sulfites.

Keeping a food diary can be a very useful tool, as it allows one to keep track of meals and any subsequent asthma symptoms, which can help identify specific triggers.

An effective way to identify food triggers is through the elimination diet, which entails cutting out suspected trigger foods from the diet for a while and then reintroducing them one at a time while keeping an eye out for reactions. For instance, if dairy is suspected, it can be cut out for two weeks before reintroducing it; if symptoms of asthma recur, dairy is probably a trigger and should be avoided. This method sheds light on how particular foods affect asthma.

The process of identifying food triggers can be further refined by consulting with healthcare professionals, such as dietitians or allergists. These professionals can conduct tests or offer guidance on safely eliminating and reintroducing foods.

Personalized advice can guarantee that people maintain a nutritious and balanced diet while avoiding foods that aggravate symptoms of asthma. People can greatly reduce the frequency and severity of asthma attacks by identifying and avoiding their personal food triggers.

CREATING REASONABLE DIETARY OBJECTIVES

The long-term management of asthma through diet requires setting realistic dietary goals. SMART (specific, measurable, achievable, relevant, and time-bound) goals are those that have a clear target and a timeline, such as increasing fruit and vegetable intake to five servings per day within a month. This goal makes it easier to monitor progress and maintain motivation.

Rather than completely overhauling the diet all at once, it's important to start with small, manageable changes. Adding a serving of fatty fish or leafy greens per week, for example, can help make the transition easier and more sustainable.

Over time, these small changes add up to significant improvements in diet and asthma management without feeling overwhelming.

A sustainable plan that supports an individual's asthma management and overall well-being can be created by setting realistic and achievable dietary goals, celebrating small victories like successfully eliminating a trigger food or consistently meeting hydration goals, and regularly reviewing dietary habits and their impact on asthma symptoms. Monitoring progress and making necessary adjustments are also essential.

ADVANTAGES OF REGULARLY EATING HEALTHFULLY

For those who suffer from asthma, eating a healthy, balanced diet has many advantages. Eating foods high in nutrients can help to lower inflammation, boost immunity, and preserve respiratory health.

 Diets high in fruits, vegetables, whole grains, lean meats, and healthy fats supply vital nutrients that improve lung function and lessen the frequency and intensity of asthma attacks.

Improved energy and general well-being are two more major advantages of healthy eating: stable blood sugar levels prevent energy crashes and increase physical endurance; for people with asthma, higher energy levels can lead to more active lifestyles, which can improve lung capacity and lessen symptoms; regular healthy eating also helps with weight management, which is important because being overweight exacerbates asthma symptoms.

The benefits of consistent healthy eating extend beyond asthma management, promoting a healthier, more balanced life. In addition, adopting a healthy diet can have positive long-term effects on mental health. Emotional stability and brain function are supported by proper nutrition, which helps to reduce stress and anxiety, which are known asthma triggers. Additionally, the sense of empowerment and control that comes from managing asthma through diet can also contribute to better mental health.

CHAPTER TWO

CRUCIAL ELEMENTS FOR MANAGING ASTHMA

FATTY ACIDS OMEGA-3

Because of their anti-inflammatory qualities, omega-3 fatty acids are critical for managing asthma. These good fats, which can be found in foods like walnuts, chia seeds, and flaxseeds, can help reduce airway inflammation, which is a common problem for asthmatics. Adding a serving of fish to your meals a few times a week or sprinkling flaxseeds on your yogurt or morning cereal can be easy ways to incorporate omega-3-rich foods into your diet.

When choosing supplements, look for high-quality options with a good balance of EPA and DHA, the most beneficial types of omega-3s. Always consult with a healthcare provider before starting any new supplement regimen to ensure it's appropriate for your specific health needs. If you have dietary restrictions that limit your intake of fish, you may want to consider using fish oil supplements to get the maximum benefit from omega-3s.

You can also incorporate omega-3 fatty acids into your diet by following some delicious recipes, such as chia seed pudding or a walnut and flaxseed smoothie; these recipes will help you maintain a consistent intake of these important nutrients while also adding some variety to your meals. As always, balancing your diet with a variety of omega-3 sources will help maximize your asthma-managing benefits.

VITAMINS AND ANTIOXIDANTS

The lungs are particularly vulnerable to oxidative stress and inflammation, which can worsen asthma symptoms. Antioxidant-rich foods like berries, leafy greens, and bell peppers should be a regular part of your diet. Vitamins like C and E, which are found in citrus fruits, nuts, and seeds, are especially helpful in lowering inflammation of the airways and enhancing lung function.

It's easy to include these high-antioxidant foods in your meals. For breakfast, try a berry smoothie that contains blueberries, strawberries, and a handful of spinach. For lunch, try a vibrant salad that includes bell peppers, kale, and a citrus dressing to increase your vitamin intake. Snacks, such as almond or sunflower seed clusters, are an easy way to get extra vitamin E throughout the day.

For an added nutritional boost, think about incorporating a range of creatively prepared vegetables into your diet. For example, you can add roasted bell peppers, steamed broccoli, and sautéed spinach to a lot of different dishes and still get a good dose of antioxidants and vitamins, which are important for managing asthma as well as general health and well-being.

MAGNESIUM AND SELENIUM ARE MINERALS

Selenium, found in Brazil nuts, eggs, and whole grains, functions as a potent antioxidant to protect lung tissue and enhance immune function; foods high in magnesium, such as spinach, pumpkin seeds, and black beans, should be regularly included in your diet. Magnesium and selenium are essential minerals for managing asthma because they help relax the bronchial muscles and reduce inflammation.

Start your day with a hearty breakfast of oatmeal with pumpkin seeds and a handful of spinach in your morning smoothie to get your magnesium and selenium intake up. For lunch, try a black bean salad with a variety of colorful vegetables to get a good dose of magnesium, and for dinner, try grilled chicken with steamed broccoli and a side of quinoa to make sure you get enough selenium.

Brazil nuts are a great way to increase your selenium intake because you only need to eat one or two nuts per day to meet your daily requirements. Eating foods high in nutrients can help manage asthma and promote overall health because they provide your body with the essential minerals it needs for various physiological functions.

A balanced diet that includes whole grains and fiber can help manage asthma symptoms indirectly by lowering inflammation and promoting better respiratory health. Whole grains, such as quinoa, brown rice, and oats, are good sources of dietary fiber, and eating a range of these grains can help you stay at a healthy weight and lower your chance of developing other inflammatory conditions.

Start your day with a high-fiber breakfast, such as oatmeal with fresh fruit and chia seeds on top. A satisfying and nutritious lunch option can be a quinoa salad with mixed vegetables and a light vinaigrette. For dinner, try whole grain wraps or sandwiches with lots of vegetables and lean proteins.

Fiber can also be easily incorporated into snacks. Try whole-grain crackers with hummus or an apple with a side of whole-grain granola. These choices not only reduce inflammation and help manage symptoms of asthma but also support digestive health in general and provide long-lasting energy.

HYDRATION: WATER IS ESSENTIAL

Drinking plenty of water throughout the day can thin the mucus in your lungs, making it easier to breathe and reducing the severity of asthma symptoms. Aim to drink at least 8 cups of water daily, more if you're active or in a hot climate. Maintaining adequate hydration is essential for managing asthma, as it helps keep the mucous membranes in the airways moist and reduces the likelihood of asthma attacks.

Apart from plain water, other hydrating options include herbal teas, coconut water, and water-rich fruits and vegetables such as oranges, melons, and cucumbers; these foods not only meet your hydration needs but also supply vital vitamins and minerals that promote overall health; it's also crucial to stay away from sugary and caffeinated drinks, as they can worsen asthma symptoms and cause dehydration.

It's easy to manage your asthma and support your respiratory health if you keep a water bottle with you at all times and set reminders to drink frequently. You can also incorporate hydration breaks into your daily routine, especially before and after exercise, to maintain optimal hydration levels.

CHAPTER THREE

TYPICAL ALLERGENS

To effectively manage their asthma, people with asthma should be especially aware of common allergens in their diet, as these can either trigger or exacerbate symptoms. Common food allergens include dairy products, eggs, nuts, wheat, soy, and shellfish. By eliminating these allergens from their diet, asthma sufferers can reduce inflammation and improve their respiratory health.

When shopping, look for allergen-free alternatives and choose whole foods that are less likely to contain hidden allergens. Cooking at home can also help control what goes into your food, ensuring it is free from potential triggers.

Carefully reading food labels is essential for avoiding hidden allergens. Many processed foods contain traces of common allergens, even if they are not obvious from the product name.

Choose restaurants that are known for their allergy-friendly menus and practices. If you have a severe allergy, always carry an epinephrine auto-injector and teach those around you how to use it in an emergency. When dining out, exercise extra caution because there is a risk of cross-contamination in restaurant kitchens.

FOODS AND ADDITIVES PROCESSED

Ingredients like sulfites, which are used in many packaged foods and beverages, can cause breathing difficulties and asthma attacks. Other additives, like artificial colorings and flavorings, can also contribute to respiratory issues and should be avoided by asthma sufferers. Processed foods are often loaded with preservatives and additives that can exacerbate symptoms of asthma.

Cooking from scratch gives you control over the ingredients in your meals, reducing the risk of consuming additives that may exacerbate asthma symptoms. Homemade meals are not only healthier but also provide better nutrition, which can strengthen the immune system and improve overall respiratory health. If you want to reduce your exposure to harmful additives, concentrate on eating a diet rich in fresh, whole foods. This includes fruits, vegetables, lean proteins, and whole grains.

Reduce your intake of processed foods and focus on natural alternatives to help asthma sufferers manage their symptoms and live a healthier lifestyle. When purchasing packaged foods, choose items with few ingredients and steer clear of those with lengthy lists of chemicals and preservatives. Look for organic and natural food labels.

FOODS HIGH IN SODIUM

High-sodium foods include canned soups, processed meats, fast food, and salty snacks. Eating too much sodium can raise blood pressure and aggravate respiratory conditions, making it more difficult for asthma sufferers to breathe. High-sodium foods can exacerbate asthma symptoms by encouraging fluid retention and inflammation in the respiratory system.

Cutting back on sodium requires cooking at home, choosing lower-sodium or sodium-free packaged foods when available, flavoring food with fresh herbs and spices rather than salt, reading food labels to identify high-sodium items and avoiding them, and gradually cutting back on salt in your diet to retrain your taste buds to enjoy lower-sodium foods.

It's also critical to stay hydrated because it helps flush out excess sodium from the body. You should also drink lots of water throughout the day and steer clear of high-sodium drinks like sodas and sports drinks. You should also increase your intake of foods high in potassium, like sweet potatoes, bananas, and spinach, as potassium can help offset the effects of sodium.

SUGARY CONDIMENTS AND DRINKS

Sugary drinks and sweets have been shown to hurt asthma management by inducing inflammation and weight gain. Sugar overconsumption can result in obesity, which is a risk factor for asthma. Sugary drinks, energy drinks, and fruit juices should be avoided as they raise blood sugar levels and cause inflammation in the body.

When you're craving something sweet, go for whole fruits, which offer natural sugars along with important vitamins, minerals, and fiber. Fruits like berries, apples, and citrus are nutritious options that can satisfy your sweet tooth without the negative effects of added sugars. Healthier options include water, herbal teas, or infused water with fresh fruits and herbs. These options provide hydration without the added sugars that can worsen asthma symptoms.

Whenever you bake or make desserts, use natural sweeteners like honey, maple syrup, or stevia sparingly. These can be sweet without triggering the same inflammatory reaction that refined sugars do. You can also keep your weight in check and lessen the effect of your sweets by eating them in moderation and as occasional treats rather than as daily indulgences.

FOODS THAT INDUCE THE PRODUCTION OF MUCUS

Foods high in saturated fats, red meat, and fried foods are some of the foods that can cause an increase in mucus production, which can clog airways and worsen asthma symptoms. Dairy products, like milk, cheese, and yogurt, are common culprits that can thicken mucus and make breathing harder for asthma sufferers.

A diet high in anti-inflammatory foods, such as fruits, vegetables, and lean proteins, can help reduce mucus production. Incorporating foods with natural anti-inflammatory properties, such as ginger, garlic, and turmeric, into your meals regularly can help support respiratory health. Warm beverages, like herbal teas, can also help thin mucus and facilitate its expulsion.

Asthma sufferers can better control their mucus production and maintain clearer airways by choosing their diet carefully. Eating foods high in omega-3 fatty acids, such as salmon, flaxseeds, and walnuts, can help reduce inflammation and support overall lung function.

CHAPTER FOUR

MEAL PREPARATION AND PLANNING

WEEKLY MENUS

Knowing which foods can help lower inflammation and enhance respiratory health is the first step in developing a weekly meal plan for asthma management. Start by choosing a range of antioxidant-rich fruits and vegetables, like berries, leafy greens, and carrots, which can support lung function. Add lean proteins, like chicken, fish, and legumes that provide essential nutrients without aggravating asthma symptoms. Include whole grains, like brown rice and quinoa, which provide fiber and sustained energy, into your daily meals.

Organize your meals into four categories: breakfast, lunch, and dinner. Make sure each meal is nutritious and balanced. For breakfast, think about dishes like oatmeal with nuts and fresh fruit, or a smoothie with spinach, berries, and a dollop of protein powder. For lunch, try hearty salads with mixed greens, grilled chicken, and a light vinaigrette. For dinner, try baked salmon with quinoa and steamed vegetables. Snacks can be easy and nourishing, like a handful of mixed nuts or apple slices with almond butter.

Use a calendar or meal planning app to plan your meals and make adjustments based on what's in season or on sale. This method not only guarantees you are consuming asthma-friendly foods but also helps you save time and effort when grocery shopping and meal preparation. Consistency is key, so repeat successful meals once a week to simplify planning.

SHOPPING LISTS FOR FOODS THAT ARE GOOD FOR ASTHMA

Making an efficient shopping list starts with figuring out which essential asthma-friendly foods to include in your diet. Start by enumerating vitamin- and antioxidant-rich fruits and vegetables like apples, oranges, spinach, and broccoli; these foods can help lower inflammation and strengthen your immune system. Next, add sources of healthy fats like avocados, nuts, and olive oil; these foods can also help reduce inflammation.

Remember to include dairy or dairy alternatives that are low-fat and free of added sugars, as high-fat dairy products can occasionally exacerbate asthma symptoms.

Lean protein sources, like chicken breasts, turkey, fish, and legumes, should be added to your list. Whole grains, like oats, brown rice, and quinoa, should also be on your list for their fiber content and energy-providing qualities.

A week's worth of meals can help you avoid making many trips to the grocery store. To make your shopping list more efficient, divide items into categories like produce, dairy, meats, and grains. This will guarantee that you have everything you need to make wholesome, asthma-friendly meals, which will help you maintain your diet and better control your symptoms.

Making a detailed plan of the dishes you'll prepare and the ingredients you'll need is a great way to organize your time and make sure you always have nutritious meals available throughout the week. To get started, choose a few asthma-friendly recipes that can be easily scaled up. Recipes like vegetable stews, baked chicken, and quinoa salads work well for batch cooking because they store well and can be portioned out for multiple meals.

Make sure you have enough containers to store your prepared meals by starting your batch cooking session with all of your ingredients prepped and ready to go. You can save time and improve the efficiency of cooking by washing and chopping vegetables, marinating proteins, and measuring out grains and spices before you begin cooking. You can cook multiple servings at a time using large pots and baking sheets.

Once your meals are cooked and cooled, portion them into individual containers and label each one with the date and contents so you know exactly what you have. This way will guarantee that you always have healthy, asthma-friendly meals ready to go, minimizing the temptation to reach for less healthy options when you're pressed for time or feeling exhausted. Store them in the refrigerator for meals you'll eat within a few days, and freeze the remainder for longer storage.

SERVING SIZES AND PORTION CONTROL

Maintaining a balanced diet, particularly when managing asthma, requires an understanding of portion control and serving sizes. To begin, familiarize yourself with the recommended serving sizes for each food group. For example, a serving of lean protein, such as fish or chicken, should be about the size of your palm; a serving of vegetables should fill half of your plate; and a serving of grains, such as rice or pasta, should be about a quarter of your plate, or the size of your fist.

Use smaller plates and bowls to help control portion sizes. This visual trick can make your portions appear larger and help you feel fuller after eating less.

Measuring cups and a kitchen scale are helpful tools for precisely portioning foods, especially when you're first starting and getting used to serving sizes. Make sure to focus on nutrient-dense foods that are high in vitamins and minerals without being overly caloric.

Aside from helping with portion control, mindful eating techniques include taking your time, enjoying each bite, and paying attention to your body's signals of hunger and fullness. You can also prevent overeating by preparing balanced meals ahead of time and portioning them out, which will also guarantee that you're getting the right nutrients to support your asthma management.

STRESS-FREE MEAL PREPARATION

Having a clear plan can save you time and lessen the anxiety of deciding what to cook every day. To start reducing meal prep stress, set aside a specific time each week to plan your meals and create a shopping list. Select easy, healthy recipes that don't require a lot of preparation. Use tools like meal planning apps or templates to keep your plan organized.

Organize your food prep so that you can quickly put together meals throughout the week without having to start from scratch. Investing in a good set of knives and kitchen tools, such as a food processor, can also expedite your prep work and make it more enjoyable. Wash and chop vegetables, marinate proteins, and cook grains like rice or quinoa ahead of time. Store these prepped ingredients in clear, labeled containers in your refrigerator.

To lighten the load and add some fun to meal prep, involve your family in the chopping, cooking, and cleanup. This will make meal prep less stressful for you and more of a shared experience. You can also use an instant pot or slow cooker for hands-off cooking, which will cook meals while you work on other projects, cutting down on the amount of time and effort you spend in the kitchen.

SMOOTHIES PACKED WITH NUTRIENTS

Smoothies that are high in vitamins, minerals, and antioxidants are a tasty and easy way to start the day. To make a nutrient-packed smoothie, start with a base of fresh or frozen fruits like berries, bananas, or mangoes. These fruits not only add natural sweetness, but they also contain important vitamins like potassium and vitamin C. Then, add leafy greens like spinach or kale for an added nutritional boost. These greens offer fiber, folate, and antioxidants.

Protein sources like Greek yogurt, almond butter, or a plant-based protein powder can be added to boost the nutritional value even more. These ingredients not only help you feel full but also support muscle repair and energy levels throughout the morning. Superfoods like chia seeds, flaxseeds, or spirulina, which are high in fiber, protein, and omega-3 fatty acids, can also be added for added health benefits.

Blend until smooth and creamy, adding a little water, almond milk, or coconut water if necessary, then pour into a glass or travel container for a quick and nutritious breakfast alternative that will last you through the day.

BREAKFAST BOWLS MADE WHOLE GRAIN

Whole grain breakfast bowls are a filling and healthy way to start the day. They contain complex carbohydrates, fiber, and vital nutrients. To make them, start with a base of whole grains, like quinoa, barley, or oats. These grains are high in fiber and can help to stabilize blood sugar levels throughout the day. Cook the grains as directed on the package, adding milk or water for extra creaminess and flavor.

Next, top your bowl with items that enhance its taste and nutritional content. Diced apples, sliced bananas, or fresh berries offer natural sweetness and a boost of vitamins and antioxidants; add almonds, walnuts, or chia seeds for protein and healthy fats that will keep you feeling full until your next meal.

A dollop of Greek yogurt or almond milk for creaminess; for extra taste and texture, drizzle your bowl with a natural sweetener like honey or maple syrup. Whole grain breakfast bowls can be made ahead of time and refrigerated for a healthy, quick, and filling breakfast option that promotes general health and well-being.

EGG-BASED RECIPES

Egg-based dishes are a flexible and healthy way to have protein, vitamins, and minerals for a filling breakfast. To get started, make classic dishes like scrambled eggs, which you can quickly cook in a non-stick skillet with a little olive oil or butter. Whisk eggs with a little milk or water to make them fluffy, and season with salt and pepper.

Or you could make veggie omelets with bell peppers, spinach, and tomatoes; these add flavor and fiber as well as vitamins and antioxidants to your meal. Just fold the omelet over the filling and cook until the eggs are set and the vegetables are soft.

Egg-based dishes are a nutritious option that can be tailored to your taste preferences and dietary needs. For a protein-packed twist, bake eggs in muffin tins with ingredients like spinach, feta cheese, and diced ham for portable and portion-controlled breakfast muffins. These can be prepared ahead of time and stored in the refrigerator or freezer, making them a convenient option for busy mornings.

OTHER DAIRY-FREE OPTIONS

Dairy-free substitutes are a healthy choice for anyone who is lactose intolerant, vegan, or just prefers plant-based foods. Start with non-dairy milk like almond, soy, or oat milk; these are fortified with calcium, vitamin D, and other necessary nutrients and have a creamy texture and mild flavor that work well as a base for cereal, smoothies, or coffee.

Dairy-free yogurt made from coconut milk, almond milk, or soy milk is a great option for a high-protein breakfast. It comes in a variety of flavors, and you can eat it plain or top it with fresh fruit, nuts, and seeds for extra taste and texture. Probiotic yogurt also helps to support gut health and is frequently fortified with vitamins and minerals to promote overall well-being.

When making recipes like pancakes or muffins that typically call for dairy, try using almond milk instead of cow's milk and coconut oil or vegetable oil in place of butter. This will keep the recipe moist and texture-friendly while removing any dairy allergies or dietary restrictions. Dairy-free alternatives are a great option for breakfast because of their adaptability and nutritional value.

HIGH-FIBER SELECTIONS

For optimal digestive health, blood sugar regulation, and general well-being, starts with high-fiber options. Start your day with a breakfast that includes whole grains like oats, whole wheat toast, or cereal with bran flakes. These foods contain soluble fiber, which lowers cholesterol and increases feelings of fullness.

Fruits like berries, apples, or pears are a good source of insoluble fiber that aids in regular bowel movements and digestion. Vegetables like avocado, spinach, or kale can be added to omelets, smoothies, or breakfast wraps to provide additional fiber and important vitamins.

High-fiber options can be tailored to your taste preferences and dietary needs, providing a tasty and nutritious start to your day. Flaxseeds, hemp seeds, and chia seeds are great sources of fiber and can be sprinkled over yogurt, cereal, or blended into smoothies for added nutritional benefits. These seeds provide omega-3 fatty acids, protein, and antioxidants that support heart health and overall wellness.

ANTI-SWELLING SALADS

Anti-inflammatory salads are a cornerstone of an asthma-friendly diet, focusing on ingredients known for their anti-inflammatory properties. These salads often include leafy greens like spinach and kale, which are rich in vitamins C and E, known to support lung health and reduce inflammation. Adding colorful vegetables such as bell peppers, tomatoes, and cucumbers not only enhances flavor but also provides essential antioxidants like beta-carotene and quercetin, which help combat oxidative stress. Incorporating omega-3 fatty acids through ingredients like walnuts or flaxseeds further boosts the anti-inflammatory benefits. Dressings can include olive oil and lemon juice, which are both anti-inflammatory and add a refreshing zest to the salad.

FILLING SOUPS & STEWS

Warm soups and stews are nourishing and comforting choices for people who control their asthma with food.

They usually include a range of vegetables, legumes, and lean proteins like fish or chicken. Garlic and onions are frequently added for their immune-boosting and anti-inflammatory qualities. Bone broth or vegetable stock broths provide a hydrating base while adding necessary minerals. Herbs and spices like ginger and turmeric add flavor and also contribute anti-inflammatory compounds. Adding whole grains like brown rice or quinoa can add fiber and help keep blood sugar stable. These soups and stews can be made in large quantities and frozen for easy, asthma-friendly meals any time of the week.

SANDWICHES WITH LEAN PROTEIN

For those who are trying to stick to an asthma diet, lean protein sandwiches are a quick and filling choice. They usually consist of whole grain bread or wraps, which help control blood sugar levels and provide fiber. Lean proteins, like grilled chicken, turkey, or tofu, provide essential nutrients without being overly saturated, which can worsen inflammation.

Leafy greens, like spinach or arugula, add crunch and flavor while also providing essential vitamins and minerals for respiratory health. Avocado slices or hummus spreads can offer healthy fats and further reduce inflammation. Low-sodium condiments, like mustard or homemade pesto, can boost flavor without adding extra sodium.

GLUTEN-FREE SELECTIONS

Choosing naturally gluten-free whole foods ensures a varied and satisfying diet that supports healthy digestion. For example, gluten-free pasta dishes made from lentil or chickpea flour offer a protein boost while remaining gentle on the digestive system.

Lean proteins, vegetables, and healthy fats like avocado or olive oil can create balanced and nutritious meals. Baking with alternative flours like almond flour or coconut flour can yield delicious treats like muffins or pancakes that are suitable for asthma-friendly diets.

Easy and quick wraps offer a flexible and portable option for asthma-friendly meals. They usually consist of whole grain or gluten-free tortillas stuffed with a blend of lean proteins, vegetables, and flavorful spreads. Protein is provided by grilled chicken or tofu strips, and colorful veggies like bell peppers, cucumbers, and spinach add crunch and vital nutrients. Spreads like guacamole or hummus enhance flavor and contribute healthy fats and additional anti-inflammatory benefits. Herbs and spices like cilantro or cumin can be added to wraps for taste and nutritional value. These portable meals are perfect for on-the-go lifestyles and can be made ahead of time for quick and easy lunches that promote respiratory wellness.

RICH IN OMEGA-3 FISH RECIPES

You can support your asthma management goals by including omega-3-rich fish in your diet. Salmon, trout, and mackerel are excellent choices because of their high omega-3 content. Grilled salmon seasoned with herbs and a squeeze of lemon make for a simple and nutritious meal. Baking trout with olive oil, garlic, and a sprinkle of almonds adds flavor and heart-healthy fats. Mackerel pan-seared with a dash of olive oil and served with a side of steamed vegetables offers a quick but satisfying dish that supports your asthma management goals.

PLANT-BASED CUISINE

Plant-based diets can be the foundation of an asthma-friendly diet because they are high in antioxidants, vitamins, and minerals. Legumes, such as chickpeas and lentils, are high in protein and provide fiber, which is important for digestive health. A hearty lentil stew with tomatoes, carrots, and spinach is satisfying and beneficial to your respiratory health. Quinoa salads with mixed greens, avocado, and a drizzle of balsamic vinaigrette make for a nutrient-dense lunch option. For dinner, try a flavorful chickpea curry with coconut milk and turmeric, served over brown rice for a satisfying and nutritious plant-based meal full of plant-based goodness.

RECIPES FOR LOW-SODIUM POULTRY

Choosing low-sodium poultry recipes can help control symptoms of asthma by lowering triggers such as excessive salt intake. A simple but flavorful main course is roasted chicken breast marinated in a mixture of garlic, lemon juice, and olive oil; a lean protein source without sacrificing flavor is grilled turkey tenderloins seasoned with fresh herbs and a light dusting of sea salt; and for a hearty dinner, bake chicken thighs with a variety of vegetables, such as bell peppers, zucchini, and onions, seasoned with low-sodium spices to add flavor without going overboard.

PASTA FOR ASTHMA PATIENTS

Pasta for asthma sufferers should be made from whole grains high in fiber and vital nutrients. For example, whole wheat spaghetti mixed with sautéed spinach, cherry tomatoes, and a little garlicky olive oil makes a tasty and filling meal. Brown rice pasta with grilled shrimp, basil pesto, and pine nuts is a tasty take on classic pasta dishes and is easy on the respiratory system.

SWEET VEGETABLE SIDES

Steamed broccoli florets seasoned with a dash of lemon zest and parmesan cheese make a light yet flavorful side dish to any main course. Grilled asparagus spears seasoned with garlic, olive oil, and a pinch of sea salt make a savory side dish that complements both fish and poultry dishes and contributes to a balanced asthma-friendly diet. Adding flavorful vegetable sides to your meals not only improves taste but also boosts nutritional value.

WHOLESOME SPREADS AND DIPS

To make healthy dips and spreads for an asthma-friendly diet, start with a classic hummus made from protein- and fiber-rich chickpeas blended with tahini, lemon juice, garlic, and a small amount of olive oil for a creamy texture that's ideal for dipping raw vegetables like carrots and cucumbers. Another option is avocado spread, which is made by mashing avocados with lime juice, salt, and pepper. Avocados are full of healthy fats and vitamins that support lung function overall.

Almond or cashew-based spreads are great for people who would rather not consume dairy. To make the spread, blend soaked nuts with nutritional yeast, lemon juice, and a small pinch of sea salt. Spread these on whole-grain crackers or use them as a spread on sandwiches with lean proteins like grilled chicken or turkey. Including these dips and spreads in your asthma diet will not only improve flavor but also guarantee that you are getting the essential nutrients that support respiratory health.

BLENDS OF NUTS AND SEEDS

As a good source of healthy fats, protein, and antioxidants, mixed nuts and seeds make great snacks for an asthma-friendly diet. To start, make a trail mix with almonds, walnuts, and pumpkin seeds; these nuts and seeds are high in vitamin E and magnesium, which support lung function and reduce inflammation. Finally, add a sprinkling of dried fruits, such as cranberries or apricots, for sweetness and extra vitamins.

A savory option is to roast chickpeas with olive oil and your preferred spices, like cumin or paprika. Chickpeas are a high-protein, high-fiber snack that helps with blood sugar regulation and respiratory health. You can also make a nut and seed mix with sesame, chia, and flaxseeds; these seeds are high in antioxidants and omega-3 fatty acids, which help to reduce inflammation in the airways.

You can eat these nut and seed mixes as a snack in between meals or as a topping for yogurt or salads.

FRUIT-BASED SNACKS

Fruit salad cups made with diced apples, oranges, and kiwis are a great way to make a healthy snack that is high in vitamin C, which boosts immunity and lowers the risk of respiratory infections. Another refreshing option for fruit-based snacks is to make fruit skewers with colorful berries like strawberries, blueberries, and raspberries. Berries are rich in antioxidants that help protect lung tissues from damage caused by oxidative stress.

Banana slices can also be dipped in dark chocolate and frozen for a decadent and healthful dessert. Studies have shown that flavonoids in dark chocolate can enhance lung function and mitigate symptoms of asthma. Alternatively, frozen bananas can be blended with a little almond milk and cocoa powder to make a rich and smooth chocolate banana ice cream.

These fruit snacks not only satiate sweet tooth but also offer vital nutrients that support respiratory health.

CRISPY VEGETABLE CHIPS

Vegetables like sweet potatoes, beets, and zucchini can be thinly sliced and then tossed with olive oil and sea salt before baking until crisp. Sweet potatoes are high in beta-carotene, which is converted to vitamin A and helps maintain healthy lung tissues; beet chips offer antioxidants that help reduce inflammation in the airways; and zucchini chips provide potassium for proper lung function. Crunchy veggie chips are a healthy alternative to traditional potato chips, offering fiber, vitamins, and minerals that support respiratory health.

These crunchy veggie chips are a guilt-free snack, or you can serve them with a homemade yogurt-based dip for extra protein and probiotics. Including these chips in your asthma-friendly diet guarantees you're getting essential nutrients while satisfying your cravings for crispy snacks.

Kale leaves can also be made into chips by massaging them with olive oil and seasoning them with nutritional yeast or garlic powder before baking.

FRIENDLY ENERGY BARS FOR ASTHMA

Convenient snacks that offer sustained energy and vital nutrients for respiratory health, asthma-friendly energy bars start with a bowl of rolled oats, nuts, and seeds. Oats are high in soluble fiber, which supports lung function and helps stabilize blood sugar levels. You can add a variety of dried fruits, such as dates and apricots, for additional vitamins and natural sweetness. Finally, you can add a spoonful of honey or maple syrup to bind the ingredients together without using refined sugars.

Use tahini or sunflower seed butter as a base instead of nuts for a nut-free option; these substitutes offer protein and healthy fats without causing a rash. Add antioxidants and flavor with ingredients like cocoa powder or cinnamon. Press into a baking pan and chill until solid, then cut into bars.

LOW-SUGAR SWEETS

Producing sweets that are low in sugar doesn't have to mean sacrificing flavor—instead, it's about using smart strategies and well-chosen ingredients to enhance flavor without the added sugars. To start, replace refined sugars with natural sweeteners like stevia, dates, or monk fruit sweeteners, which not only sweeten but also add nutrients. You can also try using fruits in recipes, like pureed berries, applesauce, or ripe bananas, to naturally add sweetness without raising the sugar content.

It's best to stick to recipes that use natural sweetness from ingredients rather than added sugars. Bake desserts that include naturally sweet fruits like berries or peaches. You can also make delicious fruit crisps with oats, nuts, and a small amount of honey or maple syrup for sweetness. Chia seed puddings with a hint of vanilla and cocoa powder, sweetened with agave syrup or honey, are nutrient-dense and satisfying desserts that are perfect for anyone trying to cut back on sugar without sacrificing taste.

Try blending ripe avocados with cocoa powder, a little almond milk, and agave syrup to make avocado chocolate mousse, a creamy dessert rich in antioxidants and healthy fats that is perfect for satisfying your sweet tooth without causing a sugar rush. Another option is to make yogurt popsicles, which are frozen treats made with Greek yogurt, fresh fruit puree, and honey drizzled over them. These icy treats are refreshing and low in added sugars, making them ideal for hot summer days.

DESSERTS WITHOUT DAIRY

For those who are lactose intolerant or have a dairy allergy, dairy-free desserts provide delectable options that everyone can enjoy. To begin, use plant-based milk substitutes in baking and cooking, such as almond milk, coconut milk, or oat milk; these milk add a smooth, creamy texture and mild flavor that complements most dessert recipes. For creamy desserts, such as puddings or custards, use coconut cream or cashew cream in place of heavy cream; these alternatives offer a rich texture without dairy.

Try substituting applesauce or mashed bananas for butter in recipes to add moisture and sweetness without compromising the nutritional value of your baked goods. You can also look into recipes that use nut or avocado butter to make creamy fillings or frostings for cakes and cupcakes. For example, you can blend ripe avocados with a little cocoa powder and maple syrup to make a rich, nutrient-dense chocolate frosting.

For frozen treats, try creating dairy-free ice creams with the base of coconut milk or almond milk; these can be sweetened with natural extracts like vanilla or blended with fresh fruit for extra sweetness. Alternatively, for a cool treat, make dairy-free sorbets with pureed fruits like watermelon, mangoes, or strawberries; these sorbets are naturally sweet and dairy-free, making them a satisfying and light dessert option.

Fruit-based sweets are a naturally sweet and refreshing substitute for traditional desserts. Fruits such as berries, bananas, apples, and citrus can be used in dessert recipes in a variety of ways, from fresh slices to purees and compotes. Fruits like these add natural sweetness and vibrant flavors to desserts. One easy but delicious dessert idea is to assemble colorful fruit skewers and serve them with a yogurt dip flavored with vanilla and honey.

Fruit crisps or crumbles are a great way to experiment with baking with seasonal fruits like apples or peaches. Toss sliced fruits with a little lemon juice, cinnamon, and natural sweeteners like honey or maple syrup. Top with a mixture of oats, nuts, and coconut oil for a crispy, golden topping that contrasts beautifully with the soft fruit filling. Fruit tarts are another great way to bake with fruit: make a gluten-free crust out of almond flour or oats, then fill it with creamy custard or yogurt and garnish it with fresh berries or sliced kiwi.

To make a cool, refreshing dessert, puree frozen fruits with a little water or juice to make dairy-free fruit smoothie bowls; you can also customize these bowls with your favorite fruits, nuts, and seeds, and top with agave syrup or honey for sweetness. Alternatively, puree fruits like mangoes, strawberries, or pineapples, then freeze the mixture in molds until solid. These homemade popsicles are a great treat for kids and adults alike.

GLUTEN-FREE BAKING

With gluten-free baking, people with celiac disease or gluten sensitivity can still enjoy delicious desserts without sacrificing flavor or texture. To begin, replace wheat flour in your recipes with gluten-free flour like almond flour, coconut flour, or oat flour. These flours have a nutty flavor and a moist crumb that work well in cookies, cakes, and muffins. Try different flour blends to see which one works best for you.

To replicate the structure and elasticity that gluten offers, binding agents such as guar gum or xanthan gum can be added to dessert recipes to improve texture and keep baked items from crumbling. For example, xanthan gum can be added to flour mixtures to make a stretchy dough that rises properly and maintains its shape while baking, or it can be used to make gluten-free pizza dough.

To improve the taste and nutritional value of your desserts, consider incorporating naturally gluten-free ingredients such as nuts, seeds, and dried fruits. For instance, you can make rich, flavorful, and gluten-free chewy almond flour cookies topped with dark chocolate chips or cranberries. You can also make flourless desserts, such as flourless chocolate cake, by combining cocoa powder, almond meal, eggs, and a small amount of honey or maple syrup.

HEALTHY SUBSTITUTES FOR TYPICAL DESSERTS

Discovering healthy substitutes for everyday desserts enables you to satiate your sweet tooth while providing your body with whole foods. To start, try adding nutrient-dense ingredients such as nuts, seeds, and whole grains to your dessert recipes. For instance, you can make bite-sized energy balls by blending dates, nuts, and rolled oats into a smooth mixture. These energy balls are high in fiber, protein, and natural sugars, and they make a great snack or dessert.

For example, try making homemade granola bars with rolled oats, almond butter, honey, and a combination of dried fruits and nuts. These bars are great for a quick breakfast or an afternoon pick-me-up. You can also look into recipes that use natural sweeteners like honey, maple syrup, or agave syrup instead of refined sugars. These sweeteners add sweetness without the empty calories and can be used in moderation to create delicious desserts.

When you're in the mood for chocolate, go for dark chocolate with a high cocoa content (70% or higher) rather than milk chocolate. Dark chocolate has more antioxidants and less sugar than milk chocolate, so it's a better option for chocolate desserts.

HERBAL TEAS TO TREAT ASTHMA

Herbal teas are a calming and all-natural way to manage asthma symptoms. Some herbs have anti-inflammatory qualities that can help reduce inflammation in the airways and facilitate better breathing. For example, ginger tea has been used traditionally to treat respiratory problems because of its anti-inflammatory properties, which can help reduce inflammation in the airways and alleviate asthma symptoms. Peppermint tea is a natural decongestant that helps to clear the airways and facilitate easier breathing. Finally, thyme tea has been used traditionally to treat respiratory issues because of its antimicrobial qualities, which can help fight respiratory infections that can exacerbate asthma symptoms.

Herbal teas for asthma relief can be made by first heating water to a boil, then steeping 1-2 teaspoons of dried herbs per cup of water (amounts vary depending on taste and potency).

Cover the tea during steeping to preserve the volatile oils that contain the medicinal properties. After the tea steeps, strain it and add honey (optional) or lemon (optional) to boost the vitamin C content and support respiratory health.

Drink the tea warm for the most calming effect on the airways, preferably 2-3 times a day during asthma flare-ups or as needed for symptom relief.

JUICES AND SMOOTHIES

Drinks such as smoothies and juices can be a tasty and nutrient-dense way to support the dietary management of asthma. Antioxidant- and vitamin C-rich foods like berries, citrus fruits, and leafy greens can help reduce inflammation and support lung function. For example, antioxidants like quercetin and vitamin C can help protect against oxidative stress in the lungs, and a smoothie made with spinach, berries, and a splash of almond milk can provide these nutrients. Omega-3 fatty acids, which are known for their anti-inflammatory qualities, can be beneficial for those who suffer from asthma.

Smoothies and juices that are suitable for people with asthma can be made by blending desired ingredients until they are smooth and creamy. If you would like something sweeter, you can add some honey or a few dates. Dairy-based products should be avoided if they aggravate asthma symptoms; instead, use alternatives like almond milk or coconut water for a creamy texture. Try different combinations to find flavors that you like and that will help your respiratory health. Smoothies and juices can be enjoyed as a light snack or meal replacement, as long as they complement a balanced asthma diet that focuses on reducing inflammation and supporting overall lung health.

HYDRATION TECHNIQUES

Asthma management depends on maintaining optimal lung function and minimizing the risk of dehydration, which aggravates respiratory symptoms. Water is the most hydrating beverage because it facilitates mucus thinning in the airways, which facilitates easier expulsion and clearer breathing. Herbal teas and diluted fruit juices can also help hydrate while offering additional respiratory benefits, such as lowering inflammation or supporting antioxidants. Sugary drinks and excessive caffeine should be avoided as they can cause dehydration and aggravate asthma symptoms in certain people.

Drink 8 to 10 glasses of water or herbal tea throughout the day to stay hydrated (adjust according to personal needs and activity levels). Bring a reusable water bottle with you to promote consistent hydration and guarantee that you always have access to fluids. Include foods high in water content in your diet, such as cucumber, watermelon, and oranges. Urine color is a simple way to check your level of hydration; light yellow or clear urine usually indicates sufficient hydration, while dark urine may indicate that you need to consume more fluids.

Sugary drinks, such as sodas, sweetened juices, and energy drinks, can cause blood sugar spikes that can trigger inflammatory responses in the body, including the airways. High-fructose corn syrup, a common ingredient in many sugary drinks, has been linked in some studies to increased asthma risk and severity. Instead, choose water, herbal teas, or diluted fruit juices without added sugars to help maintain stable blood sugar levels and support overall respiratory health. Reducing sugar intake can also worsen respiratory symptoms.

Read beverage labels carefully and select drinks without added sugars or artificial sweeteners. If you are craving something sweet, try making a homemade version using natural sweeteners like honey, maple syrup, or stevia in moderation. Fruit juices can be reduced in sugar content by diluting them with water while maintaining their natural flavors and nutritional value.

In addition to helping to thin mucus secretions in the airways, which makes them easier to expel and lowers the likelihood of mucus buildup that can exacerbate asthma symptoms, drinking enough water supports immune function, assisting the body in fighting off respiratory infections that can precipitate asthma flare-ups. Finally, staying hydrated maintains optimal moisture levels in the airways, which is crucial for effective oxygen exchange and respiratory efficiency, which can improve lung function.

To maximize the benefits of water for managing asthma, try to drink 8 to 10 glasses of water a day, with adjustments made for climate, physical activity, and individual needs. Keep a reusable water bottle with you to ensure that you always have access to fluids throughout the day and to encourage regular hydration habits. Opt for water instead of sugary or caffeinated beverages, as these can exacerbate asthma symptoms by dehydrating you.

CHAPTER FIVE

LIFESTYLE SUGGESTIONS FOR MANAGING ASTHMA

PHYSICAL ACTIVITY AND EXERCISE

Frequent exercise is essential for asthma management because it strengthens the respiratory muscles and improves lung function. Aerobic exercises, such as cycling, swimming, or walking, can improve cardiovascular health and lessen the severity of asthma symptoms over time.

It's important to start slowly and increase the intensity of your workouts gradually to prevent asthma attacks. Breathing exercises, such as diaphragmatic breathing or pursed lip breathing, can help regulate breathing patterns and manage symptoms.

Consistency is key to reaping the long-term benefits of physical activity in asthma management. Strength training exercises, which concentrate on the upper body and core muscles, can also benefit asthmatics by improving overall fitness and endurance. These exercises should be performed in a controlled environment with proper warm-up and cool-down routines to prevent sudden changes in breathing patterns. It's advisable to closely monitor symptoms during exercise and adjust intensity or activity as needed.

TECHNIQUES FOR REDUCING STRESS

Stress can worsen the symptoms of asthma, so it's important to include stress-reduction strategies in everyday activities. Progressive muscle relaxation, deep breathing exercises, and mindfulness meditation are good ways to reduce stress and promote relaxation. By using these strategies regularly, you can help control how your body reacts to stressors and lessen the chance that emotional stress will cause an asthma flare-up.

A regular daily schedule that includes time for relaxation and stress management is essential for maintaining optimal mental and physical health while managing asthma.

Hobbies or activities that promote relaxation, like yoga or tai chi, can also contribute to stress reduction and overall well-being. These practices not only calm the mind but also encourage gentle movement and controlled breathing, which can be beneficial for asthmatics.

THE VALUE OF SLEEP

Everyone needs quality sleep, but asthmatics especially need it because it's important for immune system function and general health. Creating a sleep-friendly environment and adhering to a regular sleep schedule can help minimize nighttime asthma symptoms, improve sleep quality, and prevent asthma attacks. Reducing caffeine and heavy meals close to bedtime, as well as establishing a calming bedtime routine, can also help improve overall health and sleep hygiene.

Prioritizing sleep as an essential part of asthma management can lead to improved daytime functioning and a better overall quality of life. Reducing exposure to allergens that may trigger nighttime asthma symptoms can be achieved by elevating the head of the bed slightly and using hypoallergenic bedding. Monitoring asthma symptoms before bedtime and using prescribed medications as directed by a healthcare provider can also aid in achieving restful sleep.

ENVIRONMENTAL STRESSORS AND PREVENTATIVE MEASURES

Effectively managing symptoms of asthma requires identifying and avoiding environmental triggers, which can include mold, dust mites, pollen, pet dander, and air pollution.

Regular cleaning schedules, the use of allergen-proof covers for pillows and mattresses, and maintaining ideal indoor humidity levels can all help minimize exposure to allergens in the home environment.

Working with a healthcare provider to develop an individualized action plan that includes strategies for avoiding triggers can significantly improve asthma management and reduce the frequency of symptoms.

Reducing exposure to environmental triggers can also be achieved by minimizing outdoor activities during high pollen or pollution days, using air purifiers with HEPA filters, and keeping windows closed during peak allergen seasons.

ESTABLISHING A NETWORK OF SUPPORT

Having a solid support network, which includes friends, family, medical professionals, and support groups, is crucial for providing both emotional and practical help in effectively managing asthma. Being transparent with loved ones about asthma triggers, symptoms, and treatment plans can enable them to offer the right kind of support during emergencies or attacks.

Educating close contacts about asthma, including how to recognize symptoms and administer emergency medications like inhalers or nebulizers, can empower them to assist during asthma flare-ups. Creating a supportive environment where asthma management is understood and accommodated can help improve overall well-being and better asthma control.

Participating in online communities or support groups for asthma can also help connect people with others going through similar struggles and offer helpful resources and information.

CHAPTER SIX

FAQS & FREQUENTLY ASKED QUESTIONS

HANDLING FLARES IN ASTHMA

Understanding triggers and taking preventative measures are key to managing asthma flares through diet. For those who have asthma, foods like dairy, processed foods, and sulfite-rich items like wine and dried fruits can aggravate symptoms. On the other hand, anti-inflammatory foods like fruits, vegetables, and omega-3 fatty acids can help reduce inflammation and lessen the frequency of asthma attacks.

To support respiratory health, it's important to maintain a balanced diet that includes foods rich in vitamin C, magnesium, and antioxidants. Remaining hydrated and keeping an eye on food reactions can also greatly assist in managing asthma flares. Speaking with a medical expert or dietitian can offer tailored advice on creating an efficient diet plan.

MODIFYING A CHILD'S DIET FOR ASTHMA

A balanced meal plan that promotes respiratory health and overall well-being is necessary when modifying a child's diet for asthma. To begin, cut out foods that may act as triggers, such as processed snacks, sugary drinks, and foods high in trans fats. Instead, incorporate nutrient-dense foods, such as fresh fruits, vegetables, lean proteins, and whole grains. These foods contain vital vitamins and minerals that support immune function and reduce inflammation. Including kids in meal preparation and planning helps them develop healthy eating habits and gives them the power to make nutritious food choices. Lastly, keeping regular meal times and promoting hydration throughout the day can help stabilize energy levels and support respiratory function in children with asthma.

HANDLING SOCIAL GATHERINGS AND DINING OUT

Eating out and socializing with asthma requires careful preparation and knowledge of potential triggers.

Before going to a social event, let the host or restaurant staff knows what you need in terms of diet; choose dishes that are grilled, steamed, or baked instead of fried, as these cooking techniques lower the amount of potentially harmful substances like trans fats. When eating out, focus on fresh salads, lean proteins, and whole-grain options; stay away from creamy sauces, processed meats, and heavily seasoned dishes that might contain allergens or irritants; carrying a small snack or allergy-safe foods can also serve as a backup plan in case there aren't enough options.

TAKING CARE OF COMMON MISCONCEPTIONS

To promote better understanding and management of asthma, it is important to address common misconceptions about diet and asthma. For example, one common misconception is that dairy products exacerbate asthma symptoms, but the impact of dairy varies among individuals; another is that removing all fats from the diet improves asthma control, but incorporating healthy fats like omega-3 fatty acids can actually support respiratory health; and finally, knowing that each person's specific asthma triggers can vary greatly helps in tailoring dietary recommendations to each individual's specific needs.

PROFESSIONAL HINTS AND COUNSEL

Including a variety of colorful fruits and vegetables rich in vitamins C and E, as well as magnesium and antioxidants, supports lung function and reduces inflammation. Avoiding processed foods high in additives and preservatives helps minimize exposure to potential triggers. Consulting with a registered dietitian or healthcare provider specializing in asthma can provide personalized guidance and support in developing a diet plan that meets individual needs and promotes optimal respiratory health. Expert tips and advice for managing asthma through diet focus on adopting a holistic approach to respiratory health.